Dietetic Restrictions & Recommendations in Homoeopathy

By
D.J. SUTARWALA

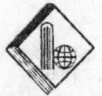

B. JAIN PUBLISHERS (P) LTD.
An ISO 9001 : 2000 Certified Company
USA — EUROPE — INDIA

DIETETIC RESTRICTIONS & RECOMMENDATIONS IN HOMOEOPATHY

Reprint Edition: 2002, 2009

All rights reserved. No part of this book may be reproduced, stored in a retrieval system or transmitted, in any form or by any means, mechanical, photocopying, recording or otherwise, without any prior written permission of the publisher.

© with the publisher

Published by Kuldeep Jain for

B. JAIN PUBLISHERS (P) LTD.
An ISO 9001 : 2000 Certified Company
1921/10, Chuna Mandi, Paharganj, New Delhi 110 055 (INDIA)
Tel.: 91-11-2358 0800, 2358 1100, 2358 1300, 2358 3100
Fax: 91-11-2358 0471 • *Email:* info@bjain.com
Website: **www.bjainbooks.com**

Printed in India by
Akash Presh

ISBN: 978-81-319-0723-8

DEDICATION
To Vanita, a source of inspiration and joy.

INTRODUCTION

An effective management of a patient, to ensure his recovery to health, is almost as important as administration of a similar medicine. All physicians would agree to the fact that an improper management in a particular case may result in slow recovery of the patient or worse, the patient's death.

Dr. S. Hahnemann, well aware of the importance of management in the treatment of sick persons, had included it as an important prerequisite for all true and judicious physicians (*vide* sec.3 of Organon of Medicine)

One can acquire the knowledge of management of disease from any of the existing classical text-books on practice of Medicine. A homoeopathic physician, however, besides this, is much more interested in the management of a sick person on an individualized basis. This is due to the fact that he knows "a man is more important than his parts".

In this compilation, I have outlined the dietetic aspect of 'Individualized Management'. The dietetic components which have an aggravating effect on the patient, while under a specific homoeopathic medicine, are to be restricted, as far as possible, keeping the individuality and the susceptibility of the patient in mind. At the same time, those dietetic components which have an ameliorating effect on the patient, are to be recommended as a means of diet. To cite an example all of us know that when *Aconite nap.* is prescribed to a patient, alcohol, sour and acidic things, fruits, vinegar etc. are to be avoided. But a very few of us would be aware of the fact that at the same time, cold drinks and cold water, coffee, milk should be recommended to that patient.

The items to be restricted and recommended are arranged in two columns against each medicine. These items are incorporated in three different grades, viz.,

'ALE' denotes Ist grade,

'Ale' denotes 2nd grade,

'ale' denotes 3rd grade.

'*', denotes, that particular item is capable of causing some ailment in a patient under the influence of the concerned medicine, e.g. in an *Abies nigra* patient, tea may produce dyspeptic symptoms and hence this is denoted by TEA*, under the 'restriction' column.

Those items which have both an aggravating and ameliorating effect under a particular medicine, are put in parenthesis '()'. While restricting or recommending these items, the physician will have to take the following things into consideration.

(1) **Patient's Susceptibility-** Whether the patient has exhibited any morbid susceptibility to that item or not.

2) **Disease of the patient -** Whether the item under question is compatible with that disease or not.

()*, denotes that particular item though does not aggravate the patient directly but it causes some ailment and as such should be restricted. eg. (alcohol) * in case of *Bryonia alba*.

In writing this compilation, I have referred and consulted:

1) Synthetic Repertory by Dr. H. Barthel & Dr. W. Klunker.

2) Repertory of the Homoeoapthic Materia Medica by Dr. J.T Kent.

3) Boenninghausen's Therapeutic pocket Book.

This compilation is offered to the noble profession with the hope that it will help physicians who have puzzled over the fact of a patient's sudden relapse when he was improving so nicely under a specific homoeopathic medicine or why a particular medicine did not work when well indicated and there being no other causes hindering patient's response.

Dr. D.J. Sutarwala

Calcutta

October 19, 1992

ACKNOWLEDGEMENTS

I would like to place on record my earnest thanks to my friend, Bimalananda Chatterjee, without whose inspiration this compilation would not have seen the light of the day.

I am also thankful to Prabir Kumar Naskar, Savita Paranjpe and Vanita Paranjpe for helping me in writing and editing this compilation. Their constant support, encouragement and inspiration made a very difficult task comparatively easy.

Dr. D.J. Sutarwala

Dietetic Restrictions and Recommendations in Homoeopathy

MEDICINES	TO BE RESTRICTED	TO BE RECOMMENDED
Abies canadensis	tea.	
Abies nigra	*tea**.	
Absinthium	bad meat	
Acetic acid	bad meat, bread and butter, cold food, sausages, spoiled sausages.	
Aconitum napellus	alcohol, beer, butter, (cold food), fatty food, fruits, hot food, pork, **SOUR AND ACIDS**, *vinegar*, sweets, warm food, (wine).	coffee, cold drinks & cold water, (cold food), milk, (WINE)
Actea racemosa	alcohol, liquor, sour and acids.	
Actea spicata	beer, spoiled fruits.	
Aesculus hippocastanum	*tea*	
Aethusa cynapium	*coffee*, MILK.	
Agaricus muscarius	*alcohol**, brandy and whisky, (coffee) cold drinks and *cold water*, cold food, dry food, stimulants, tea.	(coffee), hot food, (wine)

Dietetic Restrictions and Recommendations in Homoeopathy

MEDICINES	TO BE RESTRICTED	TO BE RECOMMENDED
Agnus castus	smell of aromatic drinks, fatty food, warm food	cold food
Allium cepa	coffee, *cucumber, spoiled fish,* peaches, bad meat, salad, warm food.	cold drinks and cold water.
Allium sativa	*cold drinks* and *cold water, meat.*	
Aloe socotrina	alcohol, *(beer) fuits, oyster,* sour and acids, vinegar.	(beer), cold drinks and cold water.
Alumina	alcohol, apples, beer, cold *drinks* and cold water, (cold food), farinaceous food, *milk,* onions, pepper, *potatoes, salt,* soup, starchy food, vegetables, vinegar, warm food, wine.	(cold food), warm drinks.
Ambra grisea	hot drinks, *hot food, milk, warm milk,* warm drinks, *warm food*	*cold drinks* and cold water, *cold food.*
Ammonium carbonicum	*alcohol,* hot drinks, *hot food,* potatoes, (sweets), warm food.	cold food, sweets
Ammonium muriaticum	alcohol, potatoes, wine.	

Dietetic Restricitions and Recommendations in Homoeopathy

MEDICINES	TO BE RESTRICTED	TO BE RECOMMENDED
Anacardium orientale	alcohol, coffee, (cold drinks and cold water), hot drinks, *hot food, warm food*	(cold drinks and cold water) *cold food*
Angustura vera	alcohol, hot food, *milk*, warm food.	cold food.
Anthracinum	eggs.	
Antimonium crudum	*alcohol, bread,* butter, *cold drinks* and *cold water, cold food,* fatty food, *fruits, sour fruits,* liquor, (milk) pancackes PASTRY, *pork,* rich food, sour and acids, stimulants, strawberries *sweets,* VINEGAR, *wine,* SOUR WINE	hot food, (milk)
Antimonium tartaricum	apples, butter, fatty food, hot drinks, hot food, milk, pork, sight of food, sour & acids, warm food, sour wine.	*cold drinks* and *cold water,* cold food.
Apis mellifica	(cold drinks and cold water), hot drinks, hot food, pickles, sour and acids, warm drinks.	(cold drinks and cold water) cold food, Milk.
Apocynum cannabinum	*cold drinks* and cold water.	warm drinks

Dietetic Restrictions and Recommendations in Homoeopathy

MEDICINES	TO BE RESTRICTED	TO BE RECOMMENDED
Aranea diadema		milk
Argentum metallicum	*milk*	coffee, sour and acids.
Argentum nitricum	*alcohol,* apples, cheese, (cold drinks and cold water), *(cold food),* fatty food, frozen food, ice*, ice-cream, meat, pastry, rich food, *(sour & acids),* sugar SWEETS, water.	(cold drinks & cold water) (cold food), (sour and acids) warm drinks.
Arnica montana	alcohol, *wine*	
Arsenicum album	ALCOHOL, apples, beans and peas, beer, *brandy* and *whisky, butter,* cabbage, cheese, *old cheese,* spoiled cheese, (coffee) *(cold drinks* and *cold water)* cold food cooked food, cucumber, *fatty food,* fish, spoiled fish, flatulent food, *frozen food,* FRUITS*, (hot food), ICE, ice-cream, liquor, *meat,* BAD MEAT, fresh meat, smell of cooked meat, melons, *(milk),* pastry, pepper, pickles, pork, raw food, rich food, salad, salt, sauerkraut	*(coffee),* (cold drinks and cold water), (cold food), hot drinks, (HOT FOOD),*(milk)* WARM DRINKS (water) (wine)

Dietetic Restrictions and Recommendations in Homoeopathy

MEDICINES	TO BE RESTRICTED	TO BE RECOMMENDED
	sausages spoiled sausages, *smell of food*, *sour* and *acids*, sweets, tea, veal, vegetables, *vinegar*, warm food, (water) (WINE) *sour wine*, *sulphurated wine*.	
Arsenicum iodatum	apples.	
Arum triphyllum	coffee, hot food.	
Asafoetida	beer, butter, *fatty food*, pork.	
Asarum europeum	ALCOHOL, hot drinks, *hot food* (warm food).	COLD DRINKS AND COLD WATER; *cold food, vinegar*, (warm food).
Asterias rubens	cider, coffee, fruits., sour and acids, sweets.	cold drinks and cold water.
Aurum metallicum	alcohol*, wine.	
Bacillinum	chicken.	
Badiaga	sweets.	
Baptisia tinctoria	beer.	

8

Dietetic Restrictions and Recommendations in Homoeopathy

MEDICINES	TO BE RESTRICTED	TO BE RECOMMENDED
Baryta carbonica	ALCOHOL, *bread*, (cold food), *hot drinks, (hot food), warm food.*	*(cold food)*, (hot food)
Belladonna	alcohol, beer, brandy and whisky, butter, coffee, *cold drinks and cold water, cold food)*, *fatty food, spoiled fish, hot drinks (hot food)* ice, liquor, bad meat, pork, salt, sausages*, *spoiled* sausages, shellfish, smell of food, *sour and acids,* sugar, (sweets), *vinegar, warm food* (wine)	cider, *(cold food)*, (hot food), (sweets), (wine), lemonade.
Bellis perennis	cold drinks and cold water, cold drinks and cold water when heated, cold food, ice*.	
Benzoicum acidum	wine.	
Berberis vulgaris	alcohol, SPOILED FISH.	
Bismuth	spices, condiments and highly seasoned food, warm food.	COLD DRINKS AND COLD WATER, cold food.
Borax veneta	alcohol, apples, *chocolate,* (cold drinks and cold water),	(cold drinks & cold water) cold food.

Dietetic Restricitions and Recommendations in Homoeopathy

MEDICINES	TO BE RESTRICTED	TO BE RECOMMENDED
	fruits, hot food, meat, mutton, pears, sour and acids, vinegar, warm food.	
Bovista	alcohol, coffee, *cold food*, dry food, liquor, wine.	hot food.
Bromium	(cold food), milk, onions, *oysters*, sour and acids.	coffee, cold drinks and cold water, (cold food), wine.
Bryonia alba	(alcohol)***BEANS & PEAS,** *beer* **BREAD,** black bread, **CABBAGE,** *old cheese,* spoiled cheese, chicken, chocolate, coffee, (cold drinks and cold water), *cold drinks and cold water in hot weather & when heated,* (cold food), *farinaceous food,* fatty food, flatulent food, frozen food, FRUITS heavy food, HOT DRINKS, *(hot food), ice,* indigestible things, *meat,* bad meat, *milk,* hot milk, oil, oysters, *pancackes, pastry,* raw food, pears, *potatoes,* rice, *Rich food,* salad, SAUERKRAUT,	(COLD DRINKS AND COLD WATER), (COLD FOOD), (hot food), vinegar, *(warm drinks),* (WATER), (wine).

Dietetic Restrictions and Recommendations in Homoeopathy

MEDICINES	TO BE RESTRICTED	TO BE RECOMMENDED
	sausages, *spoiled* sausages, starchy food, *Turnips, vegetables,* (warm drinks), WARM FOOD, (water), (wine).	
Butyricum acidum	fatty food	
Cactus Grandiflorus	*coffee,* wine.	
Cadmium sulphuratum	alcohol*, beer, cold drinks and cold water, stimulants.	
Caladium seguinum	chocolates, cold drinks and cold water, cold food, dry food, fish, pickled fish, sour and acids, vinegar.	
Calcarea arsenicosa	*alcohol,* corn meal, turnips.	
Calcarea carbonica	chocolate, *beans and peas,* brandy and whisky, cabbage, carrots, coffee, (cold drinks and cold water) (cold food), DRY FOOD, *eggs,* fatty food, flatulent food, fruits, heavy food, hot drinks, *(hot food).* indigestible things,	(cold drinks & cold water) (COLD FOOD), (hot food).

Dietetic Restrictions and Recommendations in Homoeopathy

MEDICINES	TO BE RESTRICTED	TO BE RECOMMENDED
	MILK, oysters, potatoes, rich food, *salad*, salt, *sauerkraut*, *smoked food*, sour and acids, sugar, sweets, VEAL, vegetables, warm food, water, *wine*, *champagne*.	
Calcarea caustica	beer.	
Calcarea fluorica	alcohol, cold food, eggs, fatty food, sweets.	warm drinks.
Calcarea phosphorica	*coffee*, cold drinks and cold water, *cold food*, *frozen food*, *fruits*, ice.	
Calcarea silicata	alcohol, cold drinks and cold water, cold food, (cold milk)*, wine.	
Calcarea sulphurica	MILK.	
Camphora	cold drinks and cold water, bad meat.	
Cannabis indica	alcohol, (coffee), *Liquor*.	(coffee)
Cannabis sativa		cold drinks and cold water, cold food.
Cantharis	(COFFEE), COLD DRINKS AND COLD	(coffee), (cold food), (hot food), *wine*.

12

Dietetic Restrictions and Recommendations in Homoeopathy

MEDICINES	TO BE RESTRICTED	TO BE RECOMMENDED
	WATER, (cold food), (hot food) oil, warm food, water	
Capsicum	*coffee,* hot coffee, *cold drinks and cold water,* hot food, salad.	
Carbolic acid	*alcohol,* brandy and whisky, tonics.	*cold drinks* and *cold water,* tea, *wine.*
Carbo animalis	alcohol, bread, bread and butter, cold drinks & cold water, fatty food, fish, *spoiled* FISH, meat, bad meat, milk, rich food, *decayed vegetables,* wine.	
Carboneum sulphuratum	*Alcohol,* beer, *cold food,* fatty food, fish, *(warm drinks),* warm food, wine.	(WARM DRINKS)
Carbo vegetabilis	*Alcohol*,* beans and peas, (bad brandy and whisky)*, BUTTER, *cold drinks and cold water,* cabbage, coffee, *(cold food),* (bad eggs)*, farinaceous food, FATTY FOOD* fish, *spoiled fish,* flatulent food, *frozen food,* fruits, hot drinks,	(cold food), (hot food)

Dietetic Restrictions and Recommendations in Homoeopathy

MEDICINES	TO BE RESTRICTED	TO BE RECOMMENDED
	(hot food) ICE*, (ice water)*, *liquor*, meat, *Bad meat*, pickled meat, *milk*, oysters, pastry, PORK, (poultry)*, RICH FOOD, salad, *salt**, sauerkraut shellfish, SOUR & ACIDS, *starchy food*, DECAYED VEGETABLES, *vinegar*, *warm food*, wine (bad wine)*.	
Carduus marianus	alcohol.	
Caulophyllum	coffee.	
Causticum	alcohol, *(bread)*, bread and butter, butter, chocolate, COFFEE, (cold food), *farinaceous food, fatty food; fruits, heavy food*, hot drinks, *(hot food)*, *indigestible things*, meat, *fresh meat*, pork, rich food, sour and acids, *Veal*, Vinegar, warm food.	*(bread)*, COLD DRINKS AND COLD WATER, (COLD FOOD), (hot food).
Cedron		*warm drinks*.
Chamomilla	(COFFEE), cold drinks and cold water), (cold	(coffee), (cold drinks and cold water), *(cold*

Dietetic Restrictions and Recommendations in Homoeopathy

MEDICINES	TO BE RESTRICTED	TO BE RECOMMENDED
	food), *hot drinks, (hot food, milk, sweets, tea, warm food.*	(hot food)
Chelidonium majus	*alcohol*, beer, brandy and whisky. *cold drinks* and *cold water*, cold food, *(milk)*, (warm drinks)	coffee, hot drinks, hot food, *(milk) warm milk, (warm dirnks)*, wine.
Chininum arsenicosum	eggs, fish, *fruits*, water.	
China officinalis	*alcohol**, apples, beans and peas, beer, brancy and whisky, bread, *bread and butter,* butter, *cabbage* coffee, COLD *drinks & cold water*, corn, dry food, *farinaceous food*, fatty food, fish spoiled fish, flatulent food, fruits, grapes gruel, hot food, meat, bad meat fresh meat, milk, pepper, raw food, sauerkraut, soup, sour and acids, sulphurated wine.	
Chloramphenicol	beer	
Cicuta virosa	milk.	

Dietetic Restricitions and Recommendations in Homoeopathy

MEDICINES	TO BE RESTRICTED	TO BE RECOMMENDED
Cina	bread, *mother's milk, pepper,* sweets	milk.
Cistus canadensis	coffee, sour fruits, *fruits.*	
Clematis erecta	bread, coffee, (cold drinks and cold water), hot food, pork, warm food.	(cold drinks and cold water), cold food.
Coca	*alcohol,* chocolate, *salt.*	wine.
Cocculus indicus	alcohol, beer, brandy & alcohol, beer, brandy and whisky,*coffee and, cold drinks & cold water,* cold food, smell *of food,* tea*, water.	wine
Coccus cacti	beer, *warm food,* wine.	cold drinks and cold water, cold food.
Coffea cruda	*alcohol,* bread, coffee, hot food, tea, wine*.	cold drinks and cold water.
Colchicum autumnale	alcohol, butter, coffee, *fatty food,* eggs, SMELL OF EGGS, fruits *meat, pork,* SIGHT OF FOOD, SMELL OF FOOD.	
Colocynth	beer, cheese, old cheese, (coffee), cold drinks and cold water, cold food, farinaceous	Coffee

Dietetic Restrictions and Recommendations in Homoeopathy

MEDICINES	TO BE RESTRICTED	TO BE RECOMMENDED
	food, frozen food, fruits, *oysters, potatoes, shellfish,* starchy food, wine.	
Conium maculatum	alcohol, apples, *cold drinks and cold water cold food,* MILK *(wine)*	hot food, (wine)
Corallium rubrum	wine	
Cortisone	alcohol	
Crocus sativus	cold drinks and cold water.	
Crotalus horridus	alcohol*, bread, *bad meat.*	
Croton tiglium	beer, bread, bread and butter, cold. drinks and cold water, cold food, fruits, milk, WATER.	hot milk.
Cuprum metallicum	beans and peas, bread, cabbage, (cold food), fatty food, flatulent food, heavy food, hot drinks, *hot food,* indigestible things, meat, *milk,* rich food, sauerkraut, vegetables, *warm food.*	*cold drinks* and *cold water, (cold food),* warm drinks.
Cyclamen	bread and butter, *butter,* coffee, *cold drinks* and	tea

17

Dietetic Restricitions and Recommendations in Homoeopathy

MEDICINES	TO BE RESTRICTED	TO BE RECOMMENDED
	cold water, *fatty food*, pastry, *pork*, rich food, sweets.lemonade.	
Digitalis purpurea	*alcohol**, *cold drinks* and *cold water*, cold food, *smell of food*.	tea.
Dioscorea	tea*.	
Drosera rotundifolia	butter, cold drinks and cold water, *fatty food*, pork, rich food, *salt* smell of food, sour and acids, vinegar, warm food, water.	cold food
Dulcamara	cold drinks and cold water, COLD FOOD, frozen food.	
Erigeron	beans and peas, cabbage, fatty food.	
Eupatorium perfoliatum	*alcohol*, smell of food, wine.	
Elaps corallinus	cold drinks, and cold water, cold food, fruits.	
Euphrasia	beer, butter, fatty food, spoiled fish, hot drinks, *hot food*, shell fish, *warm food*.	coffee, cold food.
Ferrum metallicum	*Alcohol, beer, butter*, COLD DRINKS AND	*(cold food)*, (milk), (tea)

18

Dietetic Restrictions and Recommendations in Homoeopathy

MEDICINES	TO BE RESTRICTED	TO BE RECOMMENDED
	COLD WATER, (cold food), dry food, EGGS, FATTY FOOD, *fruits,* sour fruits, hot drinks, hot food, *meat,* (milk) rich food, sours and acids, sweets, *(tea) vinegar,* warm food.	
Fluoricum acidum	alcohol, beer, brandy and whisky, (coffee), smell of coffee, cold food, fish, herring, melons, *peaches,* sardines, sour and acids, stimulants, sweets, tea, warm drinks, *wine,* red wine.	(coffee) cold drinks and *cold water.*
Gelsemium sempervirens	(alcohol*), (WINE)	(Alcohol), stimulants, (wine).
Glonoinum	*Alcohol,* (coffee) peaches, *(stimulants), (wine)*	(coffee), (stimulants) (wine).
Granatum	alcohol, potatoes, warm food.	
Gratiola	alcohol, coffee*, cold drinks and cold water.	
Graphites	*cold drinks* and *cold water, (cold food)* fatty	(cold food), (hott food), milk, warm milk,

Dietetic Restrictions and Recommendations in Homoeopathy

MEDICINES	TO BE RESTRICTED	TO BE RECOMMENDED
	FATTY FOOD, hot drinks, (hot food) meat, PORK, *sweets, vinegar,* (warm drinks)	milk, *warm drinks,* wine.
Haloperidol		salt.
Hamamelis virginica	fatty food, milk*, pork.	
Helleborus niger	*alcohol,* beans and peas, butter, cabbage, (cold food), *fatty food,* flatulant food, hot drinks, *(hot food),* milk, sauerkraut, *vegetables,* warm food.	(cold food), (hot food)
Hepar sulphuris-calcareum	alcohol, brandy and whisky, butter, old cheese, coffee, cold drinks and cold water, cold food, fatty food, ice, SOUR and ACIDS, sweets, tea, vinegar.	spices, condiments & highly seasoned food.
Hydrastis canadensis	alcohol,-*bread,* vegetables.	
Hyoscyamus niger	alcohol, brandy and whisky, cold drinks and cold water, *cold food,* wine	coffee
Ignatia amara	*alcohol,* beer, brandy and whisky, black bread, (COFFEE) cold	(*coffee*), *hot food,* raw food, vinegar.

20

Dietetic Restrictions and Recommendations in Homoeopathy

MEDICINES	TO BE RESTRICTED	TO BE RECOMMENDED
	drinks and cold water cold food, fruits, hot drinks, milk, spices, condiments and highly seasoned-food, stimulants, SWEETS, warm drinks, wine.	
Ipecacuanha	alcohol, butter, *coffee,* cold food, dry food, *fatty food, frozen food, fruits, sour fruits,* ice, (indigestible things),* pancackes, pastry, *Pork, rich food,* salad, smell of food, sour and acids, *sweets,* VEAL.	
Iodium	fruits, HEAVY FOOD, INDIGESTIBLE THINGS, rich food.	milk
Iris versicolor	farinaceous food, *fruits, milk.*	
Kali arsenicosum	cold drinks and cold water, cold drinks & *cold water when heated,* cold food, fatty food, ice cream, milk.	
Kali bichromicum	alcohol, -Beer*, chocolates, coffee, *cold food,* farinaceous food, fruits ice, meat, milk, *sight of food, sour and*	

Dietetic Restricitions and Recommendations in Homoeopathy

MEDICINES	TO BE RESTRICTED	TO BE RECOMMENDED
	acids, (tea).	
Kali bromatum	alcohol	
Kali carbonicum	beans and peas, *black bread*, bread, cabbage, coffee, cold drinks and cold water), *cold drinks and cold water when heated, cold drinks and cold water in hot weather,* (cold food, corn farinaceous food, fatty food, fish, *spoiled fish.* flatulent food, hot drinks, ice (hot food), meat, *fresh meat, milk, pancackes, pastry* , sight of food, soup, *vegetables, warm food.*	(cold drinks and cold water) *cold food,* (hot food.
Kali hypophosphoricum	tea.	
Kali iodatum	cold drinks and cold water, cold food, dry food, MILK, (cold milk)*.	
Kali muriaticum	beer, cold drinks and cold water, cold food, *fatty food,* pastry, rich food, spices, condiments and highly seasoned food.	

Dietetic Restrictions and Recommendations in Homoeopathy

MEDICINES	TO BE RESTRICTED	TO BE RECOMMENDED
Kali nitricum	coffee, *cold food*, fatty food, milk, VEAL*	*hot food*
Kali phosphoricum	*cold drinks and cold water*, milk, onions.	
Kali silicata	*cold drinks & cold water*, cold food, fatty food, milk.	
Kali sulphuricum	Fish.	
Kreosotum	*cold drinks and cold water, cold food*, fruits, bad meat, sour and acids, vinegar.	Hot food, warm food.
Lac caninum	milk	
Lac defloratum	MILK.	
Lachesis	ALCOHOL*, brandy and whisky, smell of coffee, cold drinks and cold water, (cold food), fish *spoiled fish (fruits) hot drinks,* hot food, *bad meat*, milk, salad, smel of food, (sour and acids), stimulants, sweets, tea, vinegar, *warm drinks,* warm food, water, *(wine)*	coffee, *(cold food)* (fruits) oysters, (sour and acids), (wine)

23

Dietetic Restrictions and Recommendations in Homoeopathy

MEDICINES	TO BE RESTRICTED	TO BE RECOMMENDED
Laurocerasus	alcohol, brandy and whisky, hot drinks, *Hot*	
Ledum palustre	alcohol*, beer, *brandy and whisky*, liquor, stimulants, *wine*.	
Lilium tigrinum	chocolate.	
Lithium carbonicum	bread, *chocolate*, fruits, tomatoes.	
Lobelia inflata	*alcohol**, cold drinks and cold water, *tea**, water.	
Lycopodium clavatum	*alcohol*, BEANS carrots, chocolate, coffee, cold drinks and cold water *(cold food)*, *dry food*, eggs, farinaceous food, *fatty food*, *fish*, *spoiled fish*, *flatulent food*, fruits, heavy food, herring, indigestible things, meat, *milk*, onions, OYSTERS, pastry, raw food, salad, salt, sardines, sauerkraut *shellfish*, sight of food, starchy food, *sweets*, turnips., vegetables, water, WINE*.	(cold food), hot drinks, HOT FOOD, warm drinks, warm food.

Dietetic Restrictions and Recommendations in Homoeopathy

MEDICINES	TO BE RESTRICTED	TO BE RECOMMENDED
Lyssin	meat, mutton, seeing or hearing water.	
Magnesia carbonica	broth, *cabbage*, (coffee), (cold food), farinaceous food, fatty food, fruits, sour fruits, heavy food, (hot food), meat, *milk**, plums, potatoes,, *vegetables,* warm food.	coffee, (cold food), (hot food), pork, salt.
Magnesia muriatica	butter (cold food), *fatty food,* fish, fruits, (hot food), meat MILK, salt, warm food, wine.	cold food, (hot food).
Magnesia phosphorica	cold drinks and cold water, cold food	
Manganum aceticum	coffee, cold drinks and cold water, *cold food.*	*Hot, warm drinks.*
Medorrhinum	brandy and whisky, meat, sweets.	
Menyanthes	bread and butter, butter, fatty food.	vinegar.
Mephitis		cold drinks and cold water.
Mercurius	*alcohol,* bread, *coffee,* cold drinks and cotr ld water, (cold food) fatty food, fruits, hot food, meat, (milk), *plums,*	*cold food*, milk

Dietetic Restricitions and Recommendations in Homoeopathy

MEDICINES	TO BE RESTRICTED	TO BE RECOMMENDED
	potatoes, *sugar sweets,* warm food, *wine, sulphurated wine.*	
Mercurius corrosivus	apples, beer, butter, eggs, fatty food, fruits, pears, potatoes, sour and acids, vinegar.	
Mercurius cyanatus	fatty food.	
Mezereum	beer, (cold food), *Hot drinks,* (hot food), warm food.	cold food, (hot food) milk, wine.
Moschus	sight of food	coffee
Muriaticum acidum	(beer), cold drinks and cold water, cold food, *fruits.*	(beer), *Hot food*
Murex purpureus	onions.	
Naja tripudians	alcohol, spices, condiments and highly seasoned food, stimulants, *wine.*	
Natrum arsenicosum	butter, cold drinks and cold water, cold food, *fatty food, fruits, milk, pork,* vinegar, *wine.*	
Natrum carbonicum	*Alcohol,* butter, *cold drinks and cold water*	BREAD

26

Dietetic Restrictions and Recommendations in Homoeopathy

MEDICINES	TO BE RESTRICTED	TO BE RECOMMENDED
	when heated, *cold drinks and cold water in hot weather,* cold food, *dry food farinaceous food,* fatty food, *fruits,* heavy food, honey, indigestible things, milk*, mother's *milk,* pears, pepper, *pork,* rich food, sour and acids, starchy food, sweets, *vegetables,* vinegar, *wine.*	
Natrum muriaticum	*alcohol,* beans and peas, *bread*,* black bread, bread and butter, butter, cabbage, coffee, *smell of coffee,* (cold food), farinaceous food, fatty food, flatulent food, herring, *Honey* (hot food), meat, *Milk,* pickles *(pork),* rich food, (salt*0 sauerkraut, smell of food, sour and acids*, vinegar, warm food, *(wine*).*	*(cold food), (hot food), (pork), (salt), (wine).*
Natrum phosphoricum	(bitter food)*, butter, cold drinks and cold water, cold food, *fatty food,* flatulent food, fruits, *milk*, sour and*	

Dietetic Restricitions and Recommendations in Homoeopathy

MEDICINES	TO BE RESTRICTED	TO BE RECOMMENDED
	acids, sugar, *sweets, vinegar.*	
Natrum Sulphuricum	apples, bread and butter, *Cabbage, coffee,* cold food, farinaceous food, fish fruits, *hot food, milk* pastry, *potatoes, rich food,* starchy food, vegetables.	
Nitricum acidum	*bread,* black bread, *bread and butter,* butter, coffee, cold drinks and cold water, *cold food,* dry food, *fatty food,* milk, *rich food, warm food.*	hot food.
Nux moschata	alcohol*, beer, (bad beer)*, *cold drinks and cold water, (cold food),* (hot food), milk*, smell of food, warm food, water	*(cold food), (hot food),* spices, condiments and highly seasoned food, *warm drinks.*
Nux vomica	alcohol*, BEER, BRANDY AND WHISKY, *bread,* black bread, bread and butter, butter, cheese, old cheese, (COFFEE*) *cold drinks & cold water,* COLD FOOD, dry food, farinaceous food, fatty food, (hot	coffee, (cold food), hot drinks, (HOT FOOD), WARM DRINKS, (wine).

Dietetic Restrictions and Recommendations in Homoeopathy

MEDICINES	TO BE RESTRICTED	TO BE RECOMMENDED
	food), *Ice*, meat, milk, onions, pepper, salad, salt, smell of food, sour and acids, SPICES CONDIMENTS AND HIGHLY SEASONED FOOD, stimulants, sweets, *tea**, veal, vinegar, warm food, (WINE).	
Oleander	bread, *fruits*.	
Onosmodium		*cold drinks and cold water*, wine.
Opium	ALCOHOL*, BRANDY AND WHISKY, (cold drinks and cold water), stimulants, (wine)	coffee, (cold drinks and cold water), cold food, vinegar, (*wine*)
Oxalicum acidum	apples, chocolate, coffee*, dry food, sour fruits, starchy food, strawberries, sugar, sweets, tomatoes, wine.	
Petroleum	*alcohol, beans and peas*, CABBAGE* dry food, FLATULENT FOOD, SAUER KRAUT, VEGETABLES, wine.	

Dietetic Restrictions and Recommendations in Homoeopathy

MEDICINES	TO BE RESTRICTED	TO BE RECOMMENDED
Phenobarbitone	fish, shellfish.	
Phosphoricum acidum	bread, *Black* bread, old cheese, spoiled cheese, *coffee, cold drinks and cold water (cold food),* dry food, *fruits, sour fruits, hot drinks, (hot food),* bad meat, spoiled sausages, sight and smell of food, sour and acids, tea, vinegar, *warm food.*	*cold food,* (hot food), milk.
Phosphorus	ALCOHOL, apples, beans and peas, (bread), black bread, bread and butter, *butter,* cabbage, cheese, cider, fatty food, fruits honey, HOT DRINKS, HOT FOOD, *milk, pastry,* rich food, SALT, SAUERKRAUT, smell of food, sour and acids, spices, condiments and highly seasoned food, sweets, tomatoes vinegar, *warm drinks,* WARM FOOD, (wine).	(bread), coffee, COLD DRINKS AND COLD WATER, COLD FOOD, frozen food, (wine).
Phytolacca decandra	alcohol, *hot drinks,* hot food., (lemonade).	cold drinks and cold water, cold food, (lemonade).

Dietetic Restrictions and Recommendations in Homoeopathy

MEDICINES	TO BE RESTRICTED	TO BE RECOMMENDED
Picricum acidum		cold drinks and cold water.
Platina	coffee.	
Plumbum metallicum	cold food, *fish*, *spoiled fish*.	*hot food.*
Podophyllum peltatum	cabbage, cooked food, fatty food, *fruits*, sour fruits, milk, *oysters*, smell of food.	
Psorinum	coffee, farinaceous food, fatty food, frozen food, *fruits, sour fruits, milk,* peaches, *sour and ACIDS.*	
Pulsatilla pratensis	*alcohol*, apples, smell of aromatic drinks, beans and peas, *beer,* brandy and whisky, BREAD, *black bread,* BREAD AND BUTTER, BUTTER buttermilk, *cabbage, chocolate, coffee,* (cold drinks and cold water), *(cold food)*, corn cucumber, *dry food eggs,* FARINACEOUS FOOD, FATTY FOOD, fish, spoiled fish, flatulant food, FROZEN FOOD	cold drinks & cold water, (COLD FOOD) (hot food) (*vinegar*)

Dietetic Restricitions and Recommendations in Homoeopathy

MEDICINES	TO BE RESTRICTED	TO BE RECOMMENDED
	FRUITS, gruel, *Heavy food*, HOT DRINKS, (*hot food*), Ice*, icecream*, indigestible things, meat,. *bad meat,melons, milk, oil onions*, oysters PANCACKES, PASTRY* plums, PORK*, *potatoes, raw food,* rice, RICH FOOD, *salad,* salt *sauerkraut,* sausages, *sour and acids, sweets,* tea, *turnips, (vinegar),* warm drinks, WARM FOOD, water, wine, SULPHURATED WINE.	
Pyrogenium	*spoiled fish,* hot drinks, *bad meat,* warm drinks.	cold food.
Ranunculus bulbosus	ALCOHOL*, *brandy and whisky, liquor,* sour and acids, vinegar, (WINE)	bacon, pork, (wine).
Ranunculus scleratus	bread	bacon, pork.
Raphanus	dry food.	
Rheum	fruits, (unripe fruits)*, plums*.	

Dietetic Restrictions and Recommendations in Homoeopathy

MEDICINES	TO BE RESTRICTED	TO BE RECOMMENDED
Rhododendron	*alcohol,* brandy and whisky, *cold drinks and cold water, (cold food), fruits*,* hot food, liquor, warm food, *wine*	(cold food)
Rhus toxicodendron	*Alcohol, beer, brandy and whisky, bread, old chese,* spoiled cheese, coffee, COLD DRINKS AND COLD WATER, *cold drinks and cold water when heated,* (COLD FOOD), spoiled fish, (hot food), ice, (ice water)*, liquor, bad meat, (milk), spoiled sausages, *sour and acids, tea,* (WARM DRINKS), *warm food,* wine.	(cold food), (HOT FOOD), (milk), (WARM DRINKS).
Rumex crispus	apples, cold food, frozen food, *fruits,* tea.	
Ruta graveolens	*Alcohol,* brandy and whisky, bread, fatty food, fruits, meat, RAW FOOD, wine.	milk.
Sabadilla	alcohol, cold drinks and cold water, cold food, smell of garlic, sight of food, water, *wine*	warm drinks, warm food.

Dietetic Restricitions and Recommendations in Homoeopathy

MEDICINES	TO BE RESTRICTED	TO BE RECOMMENDED
Sabina	milk.	
Sambucus nigra	cold drinks and cold water when heated, fruits, milk.	
Sanguinaria canadensis	*alcohol*, smell of food, sugar, sweets.	sour and acids, vinegar.
Sanicula	cheese, old cheese.	
Sarsaparilla	*bread*, cold drinks and cold water, dry food, hot food, warm drinks, warm food, wine.	cold food.
Secale cornutum	beer, bread.	
Selenium	ALCOHOL*, *fruits*, *lemonade**, liqueur, meat, salt*, sour and acids, spices, condiments and highly seasoned food, *sugar* sweets, TEA*, (*wine*).	brandy & whisky, cold drinks & cold water, (wine).
Sepia	alcohol*, apples, beans & peas, beer, *bread*, black bread, *bread and butter*, cabbage, cheese, *old cheese*, coffee, (COLD DRINKS AND COLD WATER) (cold food), *fatty food*, fish, flatulent food, *fruits*, hot drinks, *(hot food)*, meat, MILK, (boiled	

Dietetic Restrictions and Recommendations in Homoeopathy

MEDICINES	TO BE RESTRICTED	TO BE RECOMMENDED
	milk)*, onions pepper, PORK*, *potatoes, rich food*, sauerkraut, *smell of food, sour and acids*, spices, condiments and highly seasoned food, strawberries, TEA, *veal, vinegar,* warm drinks, warm food, water, sour wine, *sulphurated wine.*	
Silicea	*alcohol,* beans and peas, *beer,* cabbage, *cold drinks and cold water,* (COLD FOOD), dry food, fatty food, flatulent food, hot drinks, (hot food), meat, milk, MOTHER'S MILK, pepper, POTATOES, salt, *sight and smell of food, smoked food,* warm drinks, warm food, WINE.	(cold food), *(hot food)*
Spigelia anthelmia	*Alcohol,* brandy and whisky, *cold drinks and cold water,* (cold food) sight of food, sweets, *tea,* warm food.	(cold food), *hot food.*
Spongia tosta	*Ale,* butter, cold drinks and cold water, *fatty food,* milk, sweets, wate	warm drinks.

Dietetic Restricitions and Recommendations in Homoeopathy

MEDICINES	TO BE RESTRICTED	TO BE RECOMMENDED
Squilla	cold drinks and cold water, (cold food), hot food, sight of food, warm food.	(cold food), milk.
Stannum metallicum	beer, coffee, hot drinks, smell of food, warm drinks, warm food, water.	cold drinks and cold water, cold food.
Staphysagria	beer, bread, cheese, cold drinks and cold water, cold food, fatty food, meat, (MILK), rich food, soup, sour and acids, vinegar, wine.	(milk).
Stramonium	*alcohol,* beer, *brandy and whisky,* coffee, cold drinks and cold water, cold food, milk.	vinegar
Strontia carbonicum	alcohol, wine.	
Strophanthus hispidus	alcohol, (tea)*.	
Sulphuricum acidum	ALCOHOL, (brandy and whisky) bread, coffee, smell of coffee, *cold drinks and cold water,* (cold food), cucumber, fruits, (hot drinks), *(hot food),*	*(Brandy, whisky and wine),* (cold food), (hot food), (hot drinks).

Dietetic Restrictions and Recommendations in Homoeopathy

MEDICINES	TO BE RESTRICTED	TO BE RECOMMENDED
	milk, *oysters,* pickles, smell of food, sour and acids, vinegar, warm food.	
Sulphur	ALCOHOL*, *ale,* apples, beans and peas, *beer,* (BRANDY AND WHISKY), *bread,* black bread, bread and butter, butter, cabbage, coffee, *cold drinks and cold water, (cold food),* corn, dry food, *eggs,* farinaceous food, *fatty food,* fruits, gruel, heavy food, (hot food), indigestible things, liquor, meat, MILK, pastry, *potatoes,* rice, rich food, salads, SIGHT OF FOOD, SMELL OF FOOD, *sour and acids,* starchy food, **SUGAR,** *sweets,* turnips, veal, *vinegar, (warm drinks)* warm food, water, *(wine),* sour wine.	(cold food), *(hot food), (warm drinks),* wine).
Syphillinum	alcohol, *cold food.*	
Tabacum	alcohol.	cold drinks and cold water, cold food, vinegar.

37

Dietetic Restricitions and Recommendations in Homoeopathy

MEDICINES	TO BE RESTRICTED	TO BE RECOMMENDED
Taraxacum	*butter*, FATTY FOOD, fruits, pork, rich food.	
Tarentula Hispanica	butter, *cold drinks and cold water*, FATTY FOOD, fruits, pork.	
Terebinthina	(alcohol)*, spoiled fish, meat, shellfish.	
Teucrium marum verum	beer, bread, *cold drinks and cold water*.	
Theridion	sour fruits, meat	
Thlaspi bursa pastoris	strawberries.	
Thuja occidentalis	alcohol, apples, *beer*, butter. *coffee** (cold drinks and cold water), (cold food), *fatty food*, fish, (hot food), *onions**, pork, rich food, *smell of food*, sour and acids, stimulants, sugar, sweets*, *tea**, warm food, wine.	(cold drinks & cold water (cold food), (hot food)
Tuberculinum	smell of coffee, hot food.	
Urtica urens	fish, bad meat, *shellfish*.	
Ustilago maydis		apples.

38

Dietetic Restrictions and Recommendations in Homoeopathy

MEDICINES	TO BE RESTRICTED	TO BE RECOMMENDED
Valeriana	milk.	
Veratrum album	alcohol*, beans and peas, (beer) brandy and whisky, bread, cabbage, (cold drinks and cold water) (cold food), cucumber, farinaceous food, fatty food, flatulent food, FRUITS, grapes, (hot food), liquor, (meat), *bad meat,* pancackes, *pastry,* peaches, *pears,* pickles, *potatoes, raw food,* sauerkraut, spoiled sausages, tea, veal, vegetables, (warm drinks), warm food, wine.	*(beer)*, (cold drinks and cold water), (cold food), *(hot food)*, *(meat)*, milk, (warm drinks).
Vinca minor	coffee.	
Vipera	bad meat.	
Zincum metallicum	alcohol, brandy & whisky, bread, hot food, milk, spices, condiments & highly seasoned food, stimulants, sugar, sweets, veal, warm food, WINE.	cold drinks & cold water, cold food.
Zincum phosphoricum	bread, milk, sweets, warm drinks, WINE.	cold drinks & cold water.

Dietetic Restricitions and Recommendations in Homoeopathy

MEDICINES	TO BE RESTRICTED	TO BE RECOMMENDED
Zingiber officinale	bread*, melon*.	